The World's Fastest way to lose Weight!

By Sean Parker

Since the beginning of time,

humans have fought, loved, disagreed

agreed, fallen in love, played together,

protected and nurtured one another.

And in reflective thought I'd often

wonder which is the most powerful

aspect of human nature, physical

strength or human will power. Like

emotions of love, compared to

emotions of hate, and which one is

more potent or productive, and physical

strength has its place in history, but so

does human will power. I can recount

stories of heroism and examples of

extreme human strength like parents

lifting vehicles to rescue their trapped

children. Are soldiers using sheer will

power to survive the harsh treatment of

internment camps. So, I decided to test

them both on myself, I wondered if will

power alone could hardwire my brain

for weight loss. At that time, I was

410lbs and miserable, I tried every diet

out there, and I mean every diet, but

nothing seemed to work for me. One

day I was walking on the Levee, headed

towards the Algiers ferry, it's how I use

to exercise, I'm from Marrero Louisiana

the west bank side of New Orleans, and

I'd go walking on top the newly paved

Levee. A beautiful place to go walking

for exercise, for miles and miles it's just

evenly paved walkway, I'd park my car

two and a half miles away from the

Algiers ferry, I'd walk to the top of the

Levee, and then walk to the ferry, I did

this every day, when I'd reach the ferry,

I'd take a 30-minute rest break and then

walk back to my car, a 5 mile walk every

day, I looked at losing weight like

fighting a war, I guess a war against

obesity, or maybe against my own

laziness. But one day, as I made it back

to my car, on a particular grueling hot

summer's day, I was dripping from

sweat, head to toe, as I approached my

car, there was an older gentleman

exiting his car, "hot day young man" he

said. "Yes sir, it's burning up out here,

but at least it gives me a chance to

sweat off some of this weigh." I said

jokingly. "I lost 390lbs and I didn't even

break a sweat, not once!" the old man

said. "What?! How did you do that?" I

asked. "A year ago, I lost my wife of 40

years to cancer, devastated and

heartbroken, alone and by myself for

the first time in years, confused and a

little depressed, I guess. Emotionally I

completely shut down, and just stop

eating, I lost my appetite and zest for

life, I began to lose weight rapidly, oh,

I'd eat enough to sustain myself, but

with my wife gone, going out to dinner,

and home cooked meals, and family

dinners, all seemed pointless without

my wife, so I became sort of a recluse,

just staying home and losing weight

from not eating regular meals, I was just

so sad and emotionally withdrawn. Until

one day, it just hit me, and I realized, my

wife wouldn't want me wasting away

like this, (if she were here, she would

say stop feeling sorry for yourself, and

go forward and live your life!) And that's

just what I decided to do, I picked

myself up, and started going out again,

at first a little bit, but gradually more

and more, meeting new people,

developing new interest and enjoying

life again, that's why I'm here at the

park today, and I'm glad I bumped into

you and we had this chance to talk,

young man! I lost 390lbs in 9 months

just staying inside finding myself! So,

you don't necessarily have to work so

hard to lose weight, especially in this

summer heat, I just cut back on eating

and the weight just fell off me!" he said.

I shook the nice old guy's hand, and

thanked him for his advice, I got into my

car and head for home, thinking about

what the old guy had said me, about

controlling what you eat, and then I had

an idea just pop into my head, what if I

could change my desire for food, and

use sheer will power, to cut back on

eating?! What if every time I get hungry

my will power could take over, and

instead of eating for pleasure, I could

use will power to curve my cravings,

forgo food and seek instead more

physical stimulus, like intense bike rides

or a long swim, eating only enough to

sustain my body, like the old man did!

The next day I designed a radical new

diet program for myself, something to

test my determination to walk 5 miles

every day, combined with a search for

dramatic results! Now, remember I've

been walking 5 miles every day for 6

months, and I haven't had any

significant weight loss, a pound or two

here and there, but I couldn't keep the

weight off, I'd lose 3 pounds and then

gain 2 pounds back in a day or two, but

no real significant change in my overall

weight loss or appearance, I started at

410lbs and after 6 months I still weighed

400lbs, so, I decided to make a tactical

change to my diet plan, no more 5 mile

walks for me, I'll approach my weakness

for food, by transforming my appetite

form eating, into instant gratification for

fun instead. With satisfying fun-filled

activities, buy training my brain to crave

fun instead of food. by planning an

eventful day, to replace the feeling of

being hungry, I calculated how many

times in a day I'd get hungry, verse how

much will power I could exert during the

day to resist eating, I'd go bike riding,

play ball or go to the shooting range,

any activity that's fun, and kept my

mind off eating, from personal

observation I'd get hungry 4 to 5 times

a day, once in the morning, once

midday about 12o'clock and once in the

evening, about 7 or 8 o'clock and once

more before I'd go to bed at night, and

that was it! So every time I'd get hungry,

I'd get busy doing something fun to take

my mind off eating, for instance, if it

was late at night, I'd play video games

till bedtime, to distract my attention

from eating, earlier in the evening I'd go

visit, friends and family anything fun to

pass the time, during the day, I'd go to

the gym, and play basketball with a few

friends, whatever it took to stay active

and happy, I did whatever would keep

me on the go and busy, anything to

keep my mind off eating, I'd often wake

up 4 to 5 a.m. in the morning take a

short walk, before starting my day.

And I found staying busy keep my

thoughts off food and eating, I'd focus

on whatever task I was completing at

that time. All I know is, my will power

helps me through some extremely

tough craving attacks. Because my own

mind seemed to play tricks on me at

times, I'm serious, I would smell food

when there wasn't any cooking. Even

during my early morning ritual of

brushing my teeth washing my face,

trimming my beard, I'd smell and think

about food constantly thought-out the

day, but I didn't give in to the weakness

of the moment, even though I was

hungry, I desperately wanted to see

results, so, I toughed it out, and stayed

steady focus, and I didn't eat anything!

And after the 24 hours passed, I realized

that I could do it, will power alone is the

key to controlling my insatiable appetite

for eating, from my own inward looking

personal research, it was clear to me, I

could control my eating instead of my

eating controlling me, so, I decided to

eat one meal every other day, and

explore my appetite for something

other than eating throughout the day.

Like my cousin junie once said, "we

don't eat to get full around here, we eat

to keep from being hungry," so, my new

rule was, I'd eat only one meal on

Monday, but nothing on Tuesday, I can

eat one meal on Wednesday but

nothing on Thursday, and again one

meal on Friday but nothing on Saturday,

and one meal on Sunday, but nothing

on Monday, and on and on again. Until I

see some significant results, but I

wouldn't have to wait long, because

that first week, I lost 10lbs, I couldn't

believe what the scale was reading! I

always weigh myself first thing in the

morning, without clothing, and at the

same time every morning, and record

my results, and there was no

comparison, the results from this new

diet plan was outstanding! On the days I

can eat, I try to eat about 12 o'clock

p.m. but no later than 3 o'clock p.m.

and I'm not hungry the entire day,

because just when I get hungry at work

around 10 o'clock a.m. it's close to

launch time, and after I have eaten for

launch time, I'm usually satisfied and

full the entire day, and since I only eat

one time a day, I can choose to eat

whatever I wanted too, barbecue ribs

with steak fries, jambalaya, or red beans

and rice, seafood gumbo, boiled

crawfish and crabs, or fried chicken or

fried catfish, stuffed bell peppers

lasagna, baked macaroni and cheese or

dirty rice and potato salad. I know, but I

am from the south, and we love to eat

down here! Ask anybody, we love food!

And it's so delicious and almost

impossible to resist, and I haven't even

started on the delicacies for dessert!

But on the day's, I don't eat, I focus my

attentions on keeping busy and active

using will power to stay focused, instead

of instant gratification, that I would

normally get from eating food, every

time I got hungry I'd take a drive to my

fiancée home, and without her love,

support and encouragement, none of

this would be possible. In fact, she was

the one who suggested I get active and

try to lose weight, and I'm so thankful

for her being in my life, because this

diet is not for the faint of heart, it takes

dedication, self-reliance determination

and the unmitigated gall, to believe you

can achieve the impossible and take

control of your own life, with this diet

you have the ability to reshape your

body. My toughest challenge was the

first week, and the most grueling was

the first day without eating any food,

and it "SUCKED!!!" Going 24 hours

without eating anything, I was irritable, I

felt week and frustrated, but I stuck to

my guns and I toughed it out. The next

day I woke up, and I felt fine, in fact I

wasn't even hungry, until about 10:00

a.m. my hunger pain kick in, and I had

launch at 12 o'clock p.m. well, I had a

great big launch, I was full and satisfied

the entire day, the next day it was much

easier to get through the 24 hour

period, without eating anything, every

time I thought about food, I would put

that thought out of my mind, by taking

action and doing some fun activity, and

if I was still thinking about eating, then

that wasn't a persuasive enough way to

alter my thought patterns, I would have

to achieve a physical workout like a jog

or a weightlifting session, to make me

stop thinking about eating. And it works

every time, time after time, the

pleasure from eating when hungry is a

far greater experience, then just eating

to taste food. And the less I craved food,

the stronger my will power became to

resist craving attacks! About the fifth

day into this new diet, is when I had a

major breakthrough, my cravings for

food dropped significantly, and when I

did eat, my portions were significantly

smaller on my dinner plate, because I

was eating less food my stomach shrink

in size, and I didn't need to eat as much

food to fill full, I begin saving so much

money, I couldn't believe it, all the extra

money that I spent on fast food, was

adding up to quite a bit of money, which

lead me to conclude, I was spending

23% of my income on food, that

realization was amazing for me! Not

only I am losing weight fast, but I'm

saving money too! This seems unreal,

except for the fact, I can't eat anything

for 24-hours. Don't get me wrong, I'm

grateful I found a real solution to lose

weight, but it's not easy, my

temptations have lessened over time,

but they still exist, but I must admit, it is

easier to control my appetite, than walk

5 miles in the hot sun every day. I'd lose

a steady 5 to 10 pounds every week,

depending on if I cheated on my diet,

let's face it, we all do it, we all cheat on

our diets, even if just a little bit, but my

main focus was always to be as strict

and rigid as possible, to achieve the best

results. I started at 400lbs, and lost an

average of 5lbs a week, over the next 6

months, I lost 120lbs, and it felt great

losing all that weight, my stamina was

through the roof, my blood pressure

was in check, my clothes were falling off

me, and I had some nice clothes for a

big guy, clothes I could no longer fit,

"C'est La Vie" and I donated my favorite

gear to goodwill, but I guess that's a

small price to pay, for such awesome

results. Now standing at 6'1 280lbs and I

feel the best I have every felt in my life!

Over the next 2 months I lose another

60lbs and my weight stays a steady

220lbs, for the next year, which is my

dream size, now that I've achieved my

goal, my new battle is to maintain my

body weight. I'm sitting down to write

this in hopes of inspiring others to find

their own pathway, to lose weight

successfully. My journey was uniquely

mine, but my hope is that you as

individuals, find your own pathway to

happiness and successful permanent

weight loss, with your own uniquely

designed diet program!

<u>*GOOD LUCK OUT THERE AND GOD BLESS!*</u>